I0103475

21 DAYS OF FITNESS & FAITH

START
MOVING

A personal guide to unleashing the power of fitness in your faith

MICHELLE FRASE

Start Moving:
21 Days of Fitness & Faith

Copyright © 2025 by **Michelle Frase**

Published by **Bright Clip**

All rights reserved. No part of this publication may be reproduced, stored in a retrieval system, or transmitted in any form or by any means—electronic, mechanical, photocopy, recording, or otherwise—without prior written permission from the publisher, except for brief quotations in reviews or articles.

Unless otherwise noted, Scripture quotations are taken from either the **New International Version (NIV)**, ©1973, 1978, 1984, 2011 by Biblica, Inc.™, or the **New American Standard Bible (NASB)**, ©1960, 1962, 1963, 1968, 1971, 1972, 1973, 1975, 1977, 1995 by The Lockman Foundation. Used by permission. All rights reserved.

The scanning, uploading, and distribution of this book via the internet or via any other means without the permission of the publisher is illegal and punishable by law. Your support of the author's rights is appreciated.

Printed in the United States of America

Copyright © 2025 Michelle Frase

All rights reserved.

ISBN: 979-8-9915781-1-0

DEDICATION

To **Jesus Christ**, the One who calls me, knows me, and loves me.

Who am I?
You would speak my name. You lead my steps. You carry me. You give me breath. You traded Heaven for my cross and gave me something even better.

I am nothing without You. You have called me Yours. You sing over me. Every word in this book, every step I take, every breath in my lungs—it all belongs to You.

May this book bring glory to the only Name that saves. May my life reflect the love I never deserved but will forever praise.

It's all for You, Jesus.

CONTENTS

STOP LETTING FEAR CRIPPLE YOUR DESTINY.
LOCK EYES WITH EVERY CHALLENGE AND REMIND YOURSELF:
YOU ARE NOT DONE UNTIL YOU DECIDE YOU ARE.
IT'S TIME TO STAND UP, STEP FORWARD, AND START MOVING.

ACKNOWLEDGMENTS

First and foremost, I want to acknowledge **God**, who was moving on my behalf long before I recognized it—especially in those seasons when I was running in the opposite direction. Thank You for never giving up on me, for guiding me back to Your heart, and for showing me that every step forward is grounded in Your grace.

To my family—my children Mercy, Marya, and Everett, and my husband Vern—your love, patience, and prayers are woven into every page of this book. From the late-night brainstorms and venting sessions to the early-morning pep talks, your encouragement has kept me going on both the easy days and the hard ones. I'm forever grateful for the way you believe in my dreams and challenge me to keep growing.

To everyone moving forward with and for Christ, thank you for being a constant source of inspiration. Whether you've shared a testimony, prayed from afar, or simply walked alongside me in this journey, your support has made all the difference. Let's continue to step out in faith together, trusting that God meets us in the movement.

May this book be a testament to the power of obedience, the strength of community, and the unrelenting love of a God who calls us to keep going—no matter how many times we stumble or lose our way. And may you, the reader, find the courage to take your next bold step. It's an honor to walk this road with you.

INTRODUCTION

I remember standing in the pitch-black darkness of a Costa Rican cave, heart pounding so loudly I could barely hear the guide counting in Spanish. We had rappelled down a waterfall into the mouth of a river cave—just a small group of five, plus two local guides. One by one, we scrambled in total darkness to the top of a rocky drop-off. The plan: turn off our headlamps, edge forward, and leap into the unknown. There was a promise of water somewhere below—a hidden lake in the belly of the cave—but I couldn't see it, couldn't even hear it over the roar of my own pulse.

"Uno, dos, tres," the guide said, voice echoing off the walls. My legs locked in fear. Everything in me screamed to stay put. I tried to propel myself forward, but terror clung to my muscles. I'd never felt so vulnerable—or so aware of my own limitations. "Jump," the guide repeated, calm but firm. Time seemed to freeze. Four others had already gone, and they were waiting somewhere below. "You cannot stay here forever," another guide reminded me.

He was right. I couldn't. So I did the only thing that might move me forward: I jumped. The fall seemed endless—just pure blackness, the rush of adrenaline, and the echo of my own shout swallowed up by the cave. Then, finally: splash. Water. Relief. I turned on my headlamp and saw I'd landed safely in a subterranean lake, the faint beams of the guides' lights far above. I was wet, exhilarated, and very much alive. I swam to a small sandy ledge, breathless and amazed. The darkness hadn't changed, but my courage had. In that moment, I realized how powerful forward motion can be when every instinct is screaming for you to stay still.

I think about that cave often. There are so many reasons to stay frozen in place—fear, doubt, uncertainty. But it's movement that opens up the future.

The same is true in our faith. From the very beginning, God has called His people to move—to step forward, to trust, and to take action. Yet so often, we hesitate. We wait for a perfect moment, a clear path, or a feeling of readiness. But faith was never meant to be passive. It requires motion. It requires movement.

Over the next 21 days, we'll embark on a journey through the Old Testament—stories of ordinary people who faced impossible challenges, took leaps of faith, and discovered that God meets us when we move. You'll read about moments like Israel at the Red Sea, where God literally says, "Why are you crying out to Me? Tell the Israelites to move on!" You'll see how stepping out in obedience often precedes the miracle.

But let me be clear: this isn't just another devotional or Bible study. It's a personal guide—a challenge and a constant encouragement—for you to discover the power of movement in your spiritual and physical life. God designed us to grow deeper in faith, but He also calls us to care for our bodies, the temples He has given us. That's why we'll explore both spiritual and physical movement in these pages. We'll see how trusting God with our next step—whether it's a leap of faith, a healthier habit, or a courageous decision—can transform every part of who we are.

By the end of these 21 days, you won't just have read another book—you'll have taken real steps toward transformation. You'll have built the habit of moving forward in faith, no matter the obstacles. And you'll know deep in your soul that God meets you in the movement.

So, are you ready to move? I'm right here with you, cheering you on and reminding you that, just like in that cave, sometimes the only way to see what God has planned is to leap into the darkness and trust that He will catch you.

Then let's start moving.

1

WHY ARE YOU CRYING OUT? START MOVING!

Key Scripture: *Exodus 14:15-16*

"Then the LORD said to Moses, 'Why are you crying out to Me? Tell the Israelites to move on!'"

Standing at the Edge of the Red Sea

Picture the scene: the heat of the desert sun beating down on your neck, sweat forming on your brow, and an entire nation crowding around you—men, women, children, and the elderly, all exhausted from a frantic escape from Egypt. You look behind you and see a cloud of dust rising in the distance—Pharaoh's chariots are closing in fast, the thunder of hooves growing louder by the minute. Everyone around you is in a panic, voices rising in fear and desperation.

Then your eyes shift forward. The sight you behold sends a chill up your spine: an endless expanse of water. The Red Sea. There's no boat, no bridge, no obvious way across. The people, thousands of them, are effectively trapped. Cries of terror rise into the air: *"Were there not enough graves in Egypt that you brought us here to die?"* (Exodus 14:11)

And in the midst of this chaos stands Moses, God's chosen leader. He's the one who confronted Pharaoh. He's the one who promised the people that God would deliver them. Yet now, with an advancing army behind and a massive sea ahead, what is he supposed to do?

Moses does what we often do in moments of crisis: he cries out to God for help. But God's response is startling, almost abrupt. He doesn't say, "Stand still, I'll do everything," or "Let's talk this through." Instead, He says: "Why are you crying out to Me? Tell the Israelites to move on!"

It almost sounds insensitive—how could they move on with an ocean in front of them? But here's the core truth: God had already planned their deliverance. He didn't want them paralyzed by fear any longer. While Moses raises his staff in obedience, God parts the waters and makes a way where there was none. In that miraculous moment, the entire nation of Israel walks forward on dry ground, leaving Pharaoh's army behind for good.

What This Means for You

Let's be honest: you've probably faced your own "Red Sea" moments. Maybe you're staring at a financial crisis, a health scare, a relationship rift, or a spiritual struggle that seems to have no resolution. Behind you is the fear of past failures and regrets chasing you down. Ahead of you is an ocean of unknowns, with no clear path.

In those moments, it's natural to freeze. Fear whispers, *"This is impossible. Turn around."* Doubt hisses, *"Did God really bring you here just to watch you fail?"* You might cry out for a miracle, waiting for a dramatic rescue before you take a single step. But sometimes, God wants you to step forward before you see the sea part. Sometimes, He's already given you the command: "Why are you crying out to Me? Start moving!"

Think about that. What if the path through your problem only appears after you put one foot in front of the other? What if your deliverance is already planned, and God is waiting on you to trust Him enough to move?

Taking the First Step

This lesson isn't just spiritual—it's deeply practical, too. If you've ever started a new fitness routine or tried to change your eating habits, you know the hardest part is the beginning. You stand there, analyzing every angle, looking up workout plans or healthy recipes, but sometimes you never actually start. You're waiting for the perfect moment, the ideal conditions—much like the Israelites waiting for God to do something before they budge.

But the truth? Your body was designed to move. Waiting for perfect conditions will keep you stuck.

**The best time to begin is now,
right in the middle of your uncertainty.**

Maybe you can't see how you'll reach your goal weight, run that 5K, or improve your overall health, but your first step—however small—activates the journey. Just like God parted the Red Sea after the Israelites obeyed, you'll often see the path after you start.

Challenge

Faith Step: Identify one area of your spiritual life where you've been standing still. Maybe it's praying more consistently, joining a Bible study, or forgiving someone who hurt you. Write it down.

Today, do one thing that moves you forward in that area—like spending a focused five minutes in prayer or sending a message to reconcile with that person.

Physical Step: Think of one health or fitness change you've been putting off—maybe it's going for a walk each morning, cutting back on sugary snacks, or scheduling a doctor's appointment. Commit to starting that change today. Even a small move, like a 10-minute walk after dinner, breaks the inertia.

Sometimes, God's answer to your crisis isn't to wait— it's to move. The Red Sea might look overwhelming, but the God who parted it is the same God who leads you now. Take that step, trusting that what looks impossible to you is already possible with Him.

Your journey starts here. Will you move?

2

ABRAHAM'S FIRST STEP

Key Scripture: *Genesis 12:1-4*

"The LORD had said to Abram, 'Go from your country, your people and your father's household to the land I will show you.'"

Stepping into the Unknown

Imagine the desert wind sweeping across your face, hot and unrelenting, as you stand at the entrance of your tent. You're seventy-five years old—an age when most people are settling down, not packing up. But here you are, looking out over miles of barren landscape, with no clear destination in sight.

That's exactly where Abram stood. He was secure. He had family, possessions, a familiar routine. But then God spoke a single command that turned his world upside down: "Go." Not "Go to this city," not "Go for a short trip," but "Go from your country, your people, and your father's household to the land I will show you."

The land God would show him. In other words, God asked Abram to leave everything he knew without providing a roadmap or an itinerary—just a promise:

"I will make you into a great nation…"

Can you feel the weight of that call? Abram had every reason to hesitate. He could have demanded more details or asked God for a preview of the journey. But instead, he packed up his life and left. He didn't have all the answers, but he had enough trust in the One who called him.

What This Means for You

How often do we wait to obey God until everything makes sense? We want the whole plan laid out. We crave security, clarity, and guarantees. But the truth is, sometimes God calls us to step out first and discover the details along the way.

Maybe there's a calling on your life—something bigger than you've ever done before. It could be a change in career, a ministry opportunity, or a prompting to move to a new place. Yet you hold back, hoping God will give you a neon sign that says, "This is how it will all work out."

But that's not usually how faith works. Faith is confidence in the God who leads, not in a plan He hands us in advance. Abram didn't know where he was going, but he knew who he was following.

What about you? Is there an area where you sense God nudging you forward, yet you keep asking for a detailed map? Remember: sometimes the journey reveals itself only as you take the first step.

Trust the Process

Starting a new workout regimen or changing your diet can feel just as uncertain as stepping into an unknown land. You don't see results right away, and it's tempting to demand immediate proof: *"If I cut out sugar for a week, I'd better lose five pounds, or I'm quitting!"*

But that's not how sustainable change happens. You trust the process, commit to the journey, and let the results come in time. Like Abram leaving his home without knowing every detail, you might need to start a healthier lifestyle without instant gratification. The transformation becomes clear only as you keep moving.

Challenge

Faith Step: Think of one area where you sense God calling you out of your comfort zone—maybe it's volunteering at church, starting a small group, or switching jobs to align more with your faith. Write down what you believe God might be asking you to do. Then, take one tangible step today—send that email, fill out that application, or talk to someone who can guide you.

Physical Step: Choose one new health habit—even if it feels daunting. Maybe it's trying a new workout, meal prepping for the week, or simply drinking more water daily. Commit to it for the next seven days without worrying about immediate results. Trust that each day's consistency is leading you to a healthier future.

Remember:

**Abram didn't have a roadmap—
he had a promise.**

And that promise was enough to get him moving. The same God

who led Abram step by step is the same One who leads you now. Will you trust Him enough to take that first step into the unknown?

3

STEP INTO THE WATER

Key Scripture: *Joshua 3:13-17*

"As soon as the priests who carry the ark of the LORD—the LORD of all the earth—set foot in the Jordan, its waters flowing downstream will be cut off and stand up in a heap."

Crossing the Jordan

The sun was just beginning to rise, casting streaks of gold across the morning sky. You can almost feel the electric anticipation among the Israelite camp. Forty years in the wilderness had led them here—to the edge of the Jordan River, the last barrier before the Promised Land.

But the river was at flood stage, its waters surging with force, making it impossible to ford. The people gathered along the banks, doubt flickering in their eyes. After all this time, would they be stuck again?

Yet Joshua, their leader, gave a startling command: the priests were to carry the Ark of the Covenant—the sacred chest that symbolized God's presence—and step into the raging waters. Not wait for the water to recede. Not build a raft. But step first.

Can you imagine being one of those priests? The rushing water threatened to knock you off your feet, the roar drowning out your heartbeat. Every instinct told you to wait for safer conditions. But obedience demanded you move anyway. And the moment your feet touched the water, something miraculous happened: the current stopped flowing, and the waters stood in a heap far upstream. The riverbed turned to dry ground right beneath your feet, paving the way for the entire nation to cross.

Sometimes God calls us to move before the circumstances make sense. For Israel, the path became clear only after they stepped forward in faith.

What This Means for You

Have you ever waited for everything to fall into place before taking action? Maybe you're stuck in a cycle of "I'll do it when…"—when I have more money, when I have more time, when I'm sure it'll work out. But the truth is, faith often requires you to act first, trusting God to make a way.

That relationship you've been avoiding fixing? God might be calling you to reach out first, before you see any sign it'll resolve well. That new project at work you're hesitant to start? Maybe you need to begin, even if you don't feel fully prepared. When God nudges you forward, the key isn't to see the whole path; it's to place your foot in the water, believing He'll handle the rest.

**Miracles don't always precede obedience;
they often follow it.**

If the priests had waited for the river to part on its own, they'd still be standing there. Instead, they acted in faith, and the Jordan became a highway to the Promised Land.

Initiating the Change

Think about a time you waited for the "perfect moment" to start working out, to sign up for a gym membership, or to begin eating healthier. Perfect moments rarely exist. More often, you have to initiate the change—sign up for that class, join that walking group, or clear out junk food—before you feel entirely ready.

The Jordan River at flood stage might look like your busy schedule, your lack of motivation, or your fear of failure. If you wait for all those barriers to disappear, you might never start. But when you do take that brave step—putting on your shoes and heading out the door, choosing a healthier meal, or scheduling a workout with a friend—you'll find the path often gets clearer after you begin.

Challenge

Faith Step: Identify one situation in your life where you sense God calling you to act, but you've been waiting for a "sign" or better conditions. Write down what that step of faith looks like. Then, do something today to move forward—make the phone call, apply for the position, or reach out to that person.

Physical Step: Think of one fitness or health goal you've been postponing—maybe it's joining a local running club or cutting out sugary drinks. Start it now, even if it feels risky or too soon. Initiate the change before you see how it'll all work out.

Remember: Just like the priests had to step into the Jordan before it parted, you might need to move first, trusting God to handle what comes next. What's one step you can take today?

Your river may look dangerous, but so did the Jordan in flood season. Yet the God of the whole earth stands ready to make a way the moment you decide to step into the water.

4

STRENGTH IN THE WILDERNESS

Key Scripture: *Deuteronomy 8:2-4*

"Remember how the LORD your God led you all the way in the wilderness these forty years, to humble and test you... Your clothes did not wear out and your feet did not swell during these forty years."

Wandering, But Not Abandoned

Picture a vast desert stretching out in every direction—relentless sun, swirling dust, and the faint promise of a distant horizon. This is where the Israelites found themselves, year after year, following their dramatic escape from Egypt. It was supposed to be a short journey to the Promised Land, but instead, it turned into forty years of wilderness wandering.

At times, it must have felt endless—like an aimless trek without a finish line. Day after day, the landscape looked the same, and the people wondered if God had abandoned them. Yet, in

Deuteronomy 8, Moses reminds them: God was leading them all along. He was teaching them to rely on manna from heaven, showing them that "man does not live on bread alone" (Deuteronomy 8:3). He was allowing them to face humility and testing, all while their clothes never wore out and their feet never swelled.

In other words, even in the driest seasons, God was present, shaping their character, refining their faith, and preparing them for what was to come. The wilderness wasn't just a place they were stuck in; it was a place of transformation.

What This Means for You

Maybe you're in a wilderness of your own—a season that feels barren, like you're trudging in circles without progress. It could be a tough job situation, a lingering health issue, or a spiritual dryness that makes you question if God is still near. You might wonder, "Why am I stuck here? Where's my Promised Land?"

But here's what the Israelites' story shows us: God is still leading, even when the path seems repetitive and unfruitful. Sometimes He allows the wilderness to humble us, to show us our dependence on Him, and to strip away false securities. He's teaching us lessons we might miss if everything were easy and straightforward.

In those long, seemingly dry seasons, you can either grow resentful and give up, or you can open your heart to what God might be teaching you. The wilderness is not a waste if it shapes you into someone stronger, deeper, and more reliant on God.

Endurance in the Slow Grind

In fitness, not every day is a mountaintop achievement. Much of the time, progress is slow and unglamorous—like going to the gym on days you'd rather stay in bed or choosing a healthy meal when

17

you're craving junk food. Over the long haul, these small, consistent choices build real endurance.

Think of the wilderness as the daily grind of fitness: no overnight results, no quick fixes, just steady, faithful effort. You learn patience. You learn to listen to your body. And eventually, you look back and realize how far you've come.

Challenge

Faith Step: Identify one "wilderness" area in your life—a situation that feels dry, repetitive, or endless. Ask God to show you why you might be here and what He wants to teach you. Write down at least one insight or lesson you suspect He's shaping in you, and pray for strength to see it through.

Physical Step: Commit to one endurance-building practice this week—something that requires consistency over quick results. Maybe it's a brisk 20-minute walk each morning, steadily increasing your distance each day. Or it could be adding extra vegetables to every meal, even if you don't see an immediate payoff. Stick with it, trusting that small acts of discipline today will yield big results tomorrow.

The wilderness isn't a prison—it's a classroom.

God does some of His best work in you during these long, seemingly dry seasons. If you keep moving, keep trusting, and keep learning, you'll come out of the wilderness stronger and more prepared for the next step in your journey.

5

RUNNING WITHOUT FEAR

Key Scripture: *Isaiah 41:10*

"So do not fear, for I am with you; do not be dismayed, for I am your God. I will strengthen you and help you; I will uphold you with my righteous right hand."

Israel's Comfort in Uncertain Times

Imagine the swirling dust of an ancient road, the distant sound of approaching armies, or the faint echoes of rumors that your land might be overtaken. Such fears gripped the hearts of the Israelites during Isaiah's day. They lived under constant threat—foreign powers looming, exile a terrifying possibility. The people felt vulnerable and small, wondering if God had abandoned them to their fate.

Yet through the prophet Isaiah, God spoke a message of unshakable hope: "Do not fear, for I am with you." In a world where fear reigned, God's presence became the antidote. He promised strength for the weary, help for the overwhelmed, and a firm hand to hold them up when they felt like collapsing.

Can you picture their relief? In the midst of political turmoil and personal dread, God didn't just offer a distant, generic comfort— He offered Himself. He essentially said, "You might be afraid, but you don't have to live in that fear. I am here, and I will carry you."

This promise still rings true across the centuries. Fear might tell you to cower, to hide, or to give up. But God's voice reminds you that you're never alone—and that His strength is more powerful than whatever looms on the horizon.

What This Means for You

Fear is heavy. It weighs on your mind, saps your motivation, and keeps you from running forward in the life God has called you to. Maybe you're afraid of failure, afraid of judgment, or afraid of change. You freeze, convinced that playing it safe is better than stepping into the unknown.

But God's words in Isaiah 41:10 remind you: You don't have to carry that fear on your own. God is with you—truly, tangibly with you. His presence isn't a vague concept; it's a stabilizing reality that can calm your racing heart.

What if you lived like you believed that? What if you ran— metaphorically and literally—without the weight of fear dragging you down? You might find that the path ahead, though challenging, is far more navigable than you ever imagined.

Shedding the Weight of Fear

If you've ever tried running with a weighted vest, you know how exhausting it can be. Fear works the same way— it's like extra weight on your shoulders, making each step harder than it needs to be. But what if you laid that weight down?

In the world of fitness, fear shows up in many forms: fear of looking silly at the gym, fear of failure if you can't finish a workout, or fear of injury. These anxieties can keep you from even starting. Yet once you push past them—perhaps by doing that workout anyway or asking a friend for support—you realize how much lighter you feel. Confidence replaces dread.

The same goes for your spiritual race. The moment you decide fear won't rule you, you free yourself to run with endurance.

Challenge

Faith Step: Write down a fear that's been holding you back— maybe it's fear of sharing your faith at work, fear of taking on a leadership role at church, or fear that God won't come through in a personal struggle. Pray over that fear and visualize handing it to God. Then do something concrete that addresses that fear head- on (for example, having a spiritual conversation or volunteering for that church role).

Physical Step: What fitness goal have you avoided because of fear? Maybe it's joining a local run club, signing up for a class, or trying free weights for the first time. Commit to one action that confronts that fear—sign up for that class, ask a trainer for guidance, or invite a friend to join you.

Remember: God's promise is unwavering— "Do not fear, for I am with you." Running without fear doesn't mean your challenges disappear; it means you trust God's presence and strength more than you trust the voices telling you to stay put. Let Him carry the weight of your fears so you can move forward freely.

6

FACING THE GIANTS

Key Scripture: *1 Samuel 17*

"David said to the Philistine, 'You come against me with sword and spear and javelin, but I come against you in the name of the LORD Almighty...'"

David & Goliath—A Battle of Faith

Imagine the hush falling over the valley as two armies face each other—the Philistines on one side, the Israelites on the other. Between them stands a towering figure, nearly ten feet tall. Goliath, the Philistine champion, is covered in bronze armor that glints menacingly in the sun. His voice booms across the field, mocking Israel and demanding a challenger.

Day after day, this giant strides forward, issuing the same taunt. The Israelite soldiers shrink back in fear, certain that nobody can defeat this human mountain. Then, unexpectedly, a young shepherd named David appears on the scene. He's not a warrior—

he's there to bring food to his brothers. But when he hears Goliath's challenge, something stirs in his heart. How dare this giant defy the armies of the living God?

As David steps forward to face Goliath, the contrast couldn't be starker. Goliath is armed to the teeth; David carries only a sling and five smooth stones. Onlookers hold their breath. Surely this is a suicide mission. But David isn't relying on his own strength—he declares that he comes "in the name of the Lord Almighty." In a single motion, he slings a stone that strikes Goliath in the forehead, toppling the giant instantly. The impossible battle is won by faith.

What This Means for You

We all face giants. Maybe your giant is a deep-seated insecurity, a persistent sin, a major life decision, or a looming obstacle that feels impossible to overcome. Like Goliath, it stands before you, taunting you, reminding you of your weaknesses, and telling you to give up.

David shows us that courage isn't the absence of fear—it's trusting God's power more than we trust our own limitations. The entire Israelite army cowered because they measured the giant against themselves, but David measured the giant against God. Who could stand against the Lord Almighty?

What if you took that same perspective into your battles? Maybe you've been focusing on how big the problem is instead of how big God is. The truth is, any giant—no matter how towering—shrinks in comparison to the One who fights for you.

Courage in the Face of Intimidation

In fitness, giants show up in different forms. It might be the intimidating atmosphere of a crowded gym, the fear of injury if you push yourself too hard, or the challenge of losing a significant amount of weight. The sheer scale of the goal can paralyze you.

David's story reminds us that the size of the giant doesn't matter when your confidence is in the right place. Maybe you feel overwhelmed by how far you have to go in your health journey. But every major milestone starts with a single, confident step—knowing you don't have to do it alone. Enlist a friend or coach, rely on God's strength, and tackle your goals one "stone" at a time.

Challenge

Faith Step: Identify a "giant" in your spiritual or personal life. Is it a sin you've been battling, a financial crisis, or a relational conflict? Write it down, and then pray specifically, asking God to give you David-like courage. Share this battle with a trusted friend or mentor so you don't face it alone.

Physical Step: Think of a fitness or health goal that feels intimidating—running a 5K, overcoming a bad habit, or bench-pressing a certain weight. Set a small, tangible milestone that moves you closer to it—like running half a mile this week or lifting five pounds heavier than usual. Step up to your challenge, trusting that God is with you in every rep, every stride.

Remember: Giants fall when you face them in God's strength, not your own. Like David, you're not going into battle alone. Step forward with confidence, and watch the giant topple.

7

KEEP MOVING, EVEN WHEN YOU'RE TIRED

Key Scripture: *Exodus 17:8-13*

"When Moses' hands grew tired, they took a stone and put it under him and he sat on it. Aaron and Hur held his hands up—one on one side, one on the other—so that his hands remained steady till sunset."

Moses, Aaron, and Hur

The sun beat down mercilessly as the Israelites clashed with the Amalekites in a dry, rugged terrain. Below, soldiers fought bravely, sweat and dust mixing on their foreheads, weapons clashing in fierce combat. Joshua led the army in the valley, but high above on a hill stood Moses, staff in hand, overlooking the battlefield.

Moses knew God had promised victory, but there was a curious detail in how that victory would unfold: as long as Moses held up his hands, the Israelites had the upper hand. When his arms dropped from fatigue, the tide of battle turned against them.

At first, Moses' arms stayed steady. But as the battle wore on, weariness crept in. His muscles ached, his shoulders burned, and slowly, his arms began to fall. Panic flickered—every time his arms dipped, the Amalekites pushed forward.

That's when Aaron and Hur stepped in. Seeing Moses' exhaustion, they found a stone for him to sit on and each took a side, holding up his hands so they remained steady. Through this simple act of support, the Israelites maintained the advantage, ultimately winning the battle before sunset.

It's a vivid picture of endurance—and how sometimes, we need others to help us keep going.

What This Means for You

Life can feel like a never-ending battle at times. You start strong, confident in God's promises, but as the fight drags on—be it a long season of hardship, a demanding job, or an ongoing struggle in your family—you grow tired. Your arms begin to shake, your spirit starts to flag, and you're tempted to just let everything fall.

But Moses' story reminds us that you don't have to keep your arms raised alone. God provides community—friends, family, mentors—people who can step in when you're weary. Sometimes, endurance isn't about doing everything by yourself; it's about letting others hold you up.

Where do you need support right now? Maybe it's in prayer, maybe it's practical help like childcare or advice, or maybe it's simply an encouraging friend who can check in on you. Don't be afraid to admit your arms are tired. God's design is that we share each other's burdens.

Leaning on a Community

Have you noticed that sticking to a workout routine is easier when you have a buddy or a class to attend? There's a reason gym classes and running clubs exist: accountability. When you're tired, having someone beside you can make all the difference between quitting and pushing through.

Think of Aaron and Hur as your fitness buddies. When you can't lift your arms anymore—physically or metaphorically—they show up. This could mean a friend who meets you for an early walk so you're not tempted to skip, or a coach who guides you when you're exhausted. Leaning on others isn't weakness; it's wisdom.

Challenge

Faith Step: Identify an area where you're feeling battle-worn. It could be a prolonged season of stress, a ministry you're serving in, or a personal challenge that leaves you drained. Reach out to someone for support—ask for prayer, confess your struggle, or invite them to check in on you.

Physical Step: Don't go it alone this week. Find a workout partner or sign up for a class, group, or online community. Commit to one session where you rely on someone else's support—whether that's spotting your lifts, encouraging you on a run, or simply being there so you don't skip.

Remember: Even Moses needed help when he was weary. God didn't design you to fight your battles alone. Keep moving, even when you're tired—and allow others to help hold your arms up when you can't do it yourself.

YOU DIDN'T COME THIS FAR JUST TO COME THIS FAR. YOU'VE SHATTERED EXCUSES, SILENCED DOUBT, AND TAKEN THE FIRST STEPS WHEN FEAR TOLD YOU TO STAND STILL. THAT WAS THE BATTLE TO BEGIN—BUT NOW COMES THE WAR TO CONTINUE.

THE ENEMY DOESN'T FEAR A SPARK; HE FEARS A FIRE. AND FIRE ISN'T BUILT IN A MOMENT—IT'S FED, FANNED, AND FUELED WITH STEADY, UNWAVERING DISCIPLINE.

YOUR RED SEA MOMENTS WERE JUST THE BEGINNING. NOW, YOU BUILD. NOW, YOU STRENGTHEN. NOW, YOU ENDURE.

BECAUSE FAITH ISN'T JUST ABOUT STARTING—IT'S ABOUT FINISHING. AND THE ONES WHO FINISH? THEY REFUSE TO QUIT.

SO STAND UP. BREATHE DEEP. AND MOVE FORWARD.

STEP BY STEP. DAY BY DAY. UNTIL NOTHING CAN STOP YOU.

FROM BREAKING RESISTANCE TO BUILDING STRENGTH

You've just completed the first seven days—seven chapters that challenged you to break through resistance, push past fear, lean on community, and trust God in the face of obstacles. If you've made it this far, take a moment to breathe and recognize that you moved when it would have been easier to stand still.

- You faced your own "Red Sea" moments and took those first steps, even before the waters parted.
- You learned from Abraham's faith to obey God without having all the details.
- You stepped into the water like the priests at the Jordan, acting in faith before the miracle.
- You discovered how God uses wilderness seasons to refine you and build endurance.
- You dealt with fear, confronted giants, and remembered that even Moses needed help when he was tired.

In short, you've begun the process of getting unstuck—shaking off old excuses and patterns that held you back. That's a huge accomplishment! But the journey isn't over.

Week 2 is about building strength and consistency. If Week 1 was your breakthrough—your push to start moving—Week 2 is where you sustain the momentum. We'll dive deeper into the Old Testament, exploring stories of perseverance, daily discipline, and the steady faith that keeps you moving when the initial surge of energy fades.

Here's the key: Breaking resistance is only the first step. True transformation requires consistent, faithful effort long after the excitement wears off. Whether you're developing a new fitness habit, learning to rely on God's promises, or stepping into a new calling, discipline is what keeps you going.

Reflect & Prepare

1. **Pause and Celebrate:** What's one moment from Week 1 you're proud of? Maybe you reached out for prayer, confronted a fear, or set a small fitness goal. Write it down and thank God for the progress.
2. **Identify Your Next Hurdle:** As you move into Week 2, what's one area where you sense you'll need consistency rather than a one-time burst of effort? Keep that in mind as you enter these next chapters.
3. **Commit to Growth:** Ask God to strengthen you for the days ahead. Life won't magically slow down, and challenges might still arise. But you've already taken the hardest step—starting. Now it's time to continue in faith and discipline.

Get ready. You're about to build upon the foundation you set in Week 1, turning your breakthrough into a lifestyle of movement— both physically and spiritually. Let's continue this journey together and see what happens when we keep stepping forward, day by day, choice by choice, in faithful consistency.

Looking Ahead

In the next section, we'll explore how daily discipline, endurance, and focus can transform your walk with God and your commitment to caring for your body. You've broken through the initial walls—now it's time to strengthen the habits that will carry you the distance.

Are you ready to keep moving? Let's go.

8

STRENGTH IN THE STRUGGLE

Key Scripture: *Nehemiah 4*

"They all plotted together to come and fight against Jerusalem and stir up trouble against it. But we prayed to our God and posted a guard day and night to meet this threat." (Nehemiah 4:8-9 paraphrased)

Building the Wall Under Threat

Imagine the clamor of construction: the ring of hammers striking stone, the low rumble of oxen hauling materials, and the dusty haze of rubble all around. This is Jerusalem in the days of Nehemiah. The once-proud city walls lay in ruins after years of exile. Now, under Nehemiah's leadership, the people of God were determined to rebuild what was broken.

But progress came with fierce opposition. Surrounding enemies—like Sanballat and Tobiah—mocked and threatened the workers. They hurled insults, questioned their competence, and even plotted violent attacks. Fear and discouragement spread among the builders: What if they ambush us? What if we fail?

Yet Nehemiah refused to stop. He led the people to pray to God and post a guard day and night. Some held swords while others laid bricks; they worked with one hand on a weapon and the other on construction. Fatigue set in—"The strength of the laborers is giving out," some cried (Nehemiah 4:10). Still, they pressed on, trusting that God had called them to rebuild and would grant them success. In time, despite intimidation and weariness, the wall took shape—a testament to perseverance under relentless pressure.

What This Means for You

Life often feels like a construction zone, doesn't it? You're trying to build something worthwhile—a career, a family, a ministry, or a healthier you—while discouragement, fear, and even opposition threaten to derail you. Like the workers on Jerusalem's wall, you might have critics mocking your progress or your own self-doubt whispering, *"This is never going to work."*

Nehemiah 4 shows us that perseverance isn't about never feeling discouraged; it's about keeping going even when you do. The people prayed and took practical steps: "We prayed to our God and posted a guard day and night…" (Nehemiah 4:9). They combined faith and action, trusting that God would bless their resilience.

Where in your life are you feeling the strain of constant opposition—internal or external? Maybe it's anxiety about not being "good enough," or real people questioning whether you can succeed. Let Nehemiah's story remind you: you don't have to be fearless, you just have to keep building with one hand on faith and the other on practical diligence.

Perseverance Over Quick Fixes

In fitness, it's easy to get discouraged when results don't appear overnight. Maybe you're juggling a busy schedule, or you feel criticized by others who don't understand your goals. You might even face internal sabotage—Why bother? you might think, I'll never keep this up.

Like Nehemiah's team, you need both faith and action. You pray for strength and guidance, and then you show up consistently—whether that's taking a walk during lunch breaks, prepping healthy meals, or doing a home workout after the kids are in bed. It won't always be glamorous, but it is necessary. Over time, those consistent steps will fortify your "wall" of health, one brick at a time.

Challenge

Faith Step: Identify an area where you feel ongoing pressure—maybe a spiritual calling you've been trying to fulfill or a personal project that's stalled. Write down the sources of discouragement you're facing (critics, self-doubt, etc.). Then, pray specifically about each one, asking God for both perseverance and creative solutions to handle them.

Physical Step: Pick one fitness or health habit that has felt like a constant struggle. Perhaps you've been trying to lose weight, build muscle, or manage stress. Commit to one realistic action you can take daily—like doing 15 minutes of gentle yoga in the morning or replacing one sugary drink with water. Post a reminder where you'll see it, and consider asking a friend to "guard" this goal with you by checking in or joining you.

Remember: Progress happens in the trenches—where faith meets daily effort, and perseverance outlasts discouragement. If Nehemiah's builders could keep going with enemies threatening on every side, you can press on in your own challenges, knowing God is at work in every faithful step you take.

Progress happens in the trenches.

9

DISCIPLINED STEPS

Key Scripture: *2 Kings 5:1-14*

"Naaman went down and dipped himself in the Jordan seven times… and his flesh was restored and became clean like that of a young boy." (2 Kings 5:14)

Naaman's Seven Dips

Imagine the tension as Naaman, a respected Syrian army commander, arrives in Israel seeking a miracle. He's suffering from leprosy, a dreaded disease that isolates you from community and ravages your body over time. Word has spread that the prophet Elisha in Israel can heal the incurable—so Naaman travels with high hopes and rich gifts, expecting a grand gesture of divine power.

But when Naaman finally reaches Elisha's house, the prophet doesn't even come out to greet him. Instead, Elisha sends a messenger with a simple instruction: "Go, wash yourself seven times in the Jordan River, and your flesh will be restored." (2 Kings 5:10)

Naaman is offended. He expected a dramatic spectacle—a prophet calling on God in front of everyone, maybe waving his hand over the leprous spots. And to add insult to injury, the Jordan is neither impressive nor pristine compared to the rivers of Damascus. Furious, Naaman nearly turns around to go home.

But his servants plead with him: *If the prophet had asked you to do something difficult, wouldn't you have tried it? This is simple. Just do it.* (2 Kings 5:13 paraphrased)

Reluctantly, Naaman goes down to the muddy Jordan. He dips once. Nothing changes. Twice. Three times. Still no improvement. Seven dips Elisha said. By the seventh time, Naaman emerges completely healed—his skin restored as if brand new. Had he clung to pride or dismissed Elisha's instructions, he would have missed the miracle.

What This Means for You

Sometimes, God's path to healing or growth looks too simple or too humbling. You might think, *Surely there's a more dignified, dramatic way for God to work.* But like Naaman, we can miss out if we're too proud or impatient to follow God's instructions—especially when they seem mundane.

Naaman's story is about consistent, humble obedience. He didn't see results after the first dip, or the second, or the third. Yet he kept going, trusting the prophet's words. His breakthrough happened only after he followed through—dips 1 through 7, exactly as commanded.

Where do you need that same discipline? Maybe you're looking for a spiritual breakthrough, but God's nudging you to do something humble—like committing to daily prayer, seeking wise counsel, or reconciling with someone you've wronged. Or perhaps you're longing for healing in your emotions or finances, but the steps God gives you feel too simple. Don't let pride rob you of God's blessing.

Small, Repeated Actions Yield Big Results

In the fitness world, true transformation rarely comes from a one-time heroic effort. It's the small, repeated actions—showing up for that class every week, logging your meals daily, or doing those extra reps consistently. It might feel tedious or unimpressive at first, but each "dip in the Jordan" contributes to a bigger picture.

Like Naaman, you might not see immediate results. Maybe you work out for a week and the scale doesn't budge, or you cut sugary snacks for a month and only see minor changes. But discipline means you keep going, trusting that each step is part of your long-term success.

Challenge

Faith Step: Ask God to reveal one area in your spiritual life where simple, humble obedience is needed—maybe consistent Bible reading, regular attendance at a small group, or daily journaling your prayers. Commit to doing it daily for a set period (like seven days), resisting the urge to quit just because you don't see immediate fruit.

Physical Step: Pick a health habit that feels mundane or "too simple" but could make a difference if done consistently—like drinking a glass of water first thing in the morning, taking the stairs whenever possible, or stretching for five minutes before bed. Do it every day for a week and see if you notice any shifts in how you feel.

Remember: Naaman's miracle happened on the seventh dip, not the first. Consistency and humble obedience are often the keys that unlock transformation. Keep dipping, keep trusting, and watch what God can do.

10

KEEP YOUR EYES ON THE GOAL

Key Scripture: *Nehemiah 6:1-9*

"I am carrying on a great project and cannot go down. Why should the work stop while I leave it and go down to you?" (Nehemiah 6:3 paraphrased)

Nehemiah's Distractions

The walls of Jerusalem were rising rapidly under Nehemiah's leadership. Stones and mortar piled higher each day, hope rekindling in the hearts of the exiled Israelites who had returned to rebuild their beloved city. From a distance, their enemies watched with growing alarm.

Among them were Sanballat, Tobiah, and Geshem—leaders who had mocked and threatened Nehemiah's team from the start. But now, seeing the wall nearly complete, they changed tactics. Four times, they sent messages to Nehemiah, inviting him to a "meeting," hoping to lure him away and harm him. Nehemiah saw through the deception.

He famously replied: "I am carrying on a great project and cannot go down. Why should the work stop while I leave it and go down to you?" (Nehemiah 6:3) Despite their repeated attempts—and even rumors meant to intimidate him—Nehemiah refused to abandon his post or lose focus. He had a mission: to finish the wall. He wouldn't let distractions or fear derail him.

Before long, the wall was completed in just 52 days—an astonishing feat that left their enemies discouraged. Nehemiah's unwavering commitment and trust in God had overcome every scheme.

What This Means for You

Have you ever set a goal or felt called to a particular mission, only to find yourself bombarded by distractions, doubts, or seemingly urgent demands that pull you away? Life gets noisy—friends want your time, social media pings, side projects beckon, and even your own procrastination can feel like an irresistible invitation.

Nehemiah's story teaches us the value of laser-like focus. When God puts a calling on your heart—be it rebuilding your spiritual life, working on a marriage, or embarking on a health journey— distractions will come. Some might be innocent, others malicious, but all threaten to slow or sabotage your progress.

Staying on the wall means saying no to good things for the sake of the best thing. It means prioritizing your calling over the noise. Sometimes, like Nehemiah, you'll need to respond with unwavering clarity: *I cannot come down. My work isn't finished.*

Blocking Out the Noise

In the realm of fitness, distractions are everywhere: new diets promising overnight results, workout fads, or even well-meaning friends who say, "Skip the gym—let's grab dessert instead!" If you want to see genuine progress, you have to keep your eyes on the goal. It's easy to start strong but lose momentum when the novelty wears off or when life gets busy.

Like Nehemiah, remember why you started. What's your bigger "why"? Is it to be healthier for your family, to steward your body as God's temple, or to gain energy and confidence? Keeping that central motivation in mind helps you say no to distractions and temptations that pull you off track.

Challenge

Faith Step: Identify one crucial goal or mission God has placed on your heart. It might be developing a consistent prayer life, restoring a broken relationship, or serving in a specific ministry. Now, list two or three distractions that frequently tempt you to abandon or delay this goal. For each distraction, decide how you'll handle it—maybe setting boundaries, asking someone to hold you accountable, or turning off notifications during your prayer time.

Physical Step: Pinpoint a primary health or fitness goal for this season—like running a certain distance, adopting a consistent workout schedule, or eating more whole foods. Write down the biggest distraction(s) or excuses that typically derail you. Brainstorm one strategy to counter each distraction, such as scheduling workouts in your calendar or meal-prepping in advance.

Remember: Nehemiah finished the wall because he refused to come down, no matter how enticing or threatening the distractions seemed. Keep your eyes on the goal God has given you, and don't stop until the work is done.

11

THE STRENGTH TO STAND FIRM

Key scripture: *2 Chronicles 20:15–17*

"Do not be afraid or discouraged... for the battle is not yours, but God's." (2 chronicles 20:15 paraphrased)

Jehoshaphat's Battle

A fearsome alliance of Moabites, Ammonites, and others advanced toward Judah, determined to destroy King Jehoshaphat and his people. Overwhelmed by the size of the enemy forces, Jehoshaphat did not muster more troops or rush into negotiations. Instead, he called the nation to fast and pray, acknowledging that their hope rested solely in God's power. As the people gathered, God spoke through a prophet, assuring them that they would not need to fight in their own strength. They were to take their positions, stand firm, and watch God move on their behalf. In faithful obedience, the army of Judah placed singers and worshippers at the front of their ranks, praising God rather than trembling before the enemy. By the time they reached the battlefield, their enemies had turned on one another, leaving Judah's soldiers stunned by God's miraculous intervention. Their role had been simply to remain steadfast, trusting that the Lord would secure the victory.

What This Means for You

Jehoshaphat's story reminds us that sometimes the greatest act of faith is choosing not to spring into frantic action. When we confront situations that feel impossible—whether in our relationships, finances, or personal struggles—we often try to fix everything ourselves. Yet, there are moments when God calls us to stand firm and witness what He will do. Standing firm is not passive resignation; rather, it is an active stance of trust. It is a deliberate decision to seek God first, remain where He has placed you, and resist the urge to force an outcome in your own strength. By acknowledging that the battle ultimately belongs to the Lord, you open yourself up to God's miraculous power, just as Jehoshaphat did. Sometimes, true movement in faith comes through patience, prayer, and an unwavering commitment to follow God's lead.

Standing Strong Against Discouragement

In your fitness and health journey, the call to "stand firm" often means not giving up when results are slow or obstacles arise. Progress in exercise, weight loss, or overall wellness can stall, leading to frustration or the temptation to abandon your goals. But just as the people of Judah discovered, perseverance under pressure can yield remarkable outcomes. Standing strong in the face of discouragement means holding on to the vision of why you started and believing that consistent effort—backed by prayer and healthy habits—will eventually produce tangible results. Instead of viewing setbacks as final defeats, see them as reminders to press on, trusting that God's power works not only in your spiritual life but in every aspect of your journey.

Challenge

Faith Step: Think about a challenge in your life that feels too big to handle. Rather than trying to fix it through sheer determination, set aside intentional time each day this week to pray for God's guidance and intervention. Write down one way you will remain steadfast—maybe by reading a chapter of Scripture every morning, seeking pastoral or trusted counsel, or journaling your prayers to maintain focus on God's presence.

Physical Step: Examine a health or fitness goal you have begun but feel tempted to quit—maybe it's running a certain distance, adjusting your diet, or committing to a more active lifestyle. Determine how you can stay firm in that commitment. You might schedule workouts as non-negotiable appointments, invite a friend to join you for accountability, or plan ahead for meal prep. If discouragement arises, remind yourself that just as God delivered Judah when they stood firm, He can also strengthen you to stay the course, overcome setbacks, and see the fruit of your perseverance.

Remember that sometimes the most powerful "move" you can make is not to charge forward but to hold your ground in faith. Like Jehoshaphat and his people, trust that as you take your position and stand firm, you leave room for God's power to accomplish more than you could manage on your own.

12

RENEWED IN THE WAITING

Key Scripture: *Psalm 27:13–14*

"I remain confident of this: I will see the goodness of the LORD…
wait for the LORD; be strong and take heart and wait for the
LORD." (Psalm 27:13–14 paraphrased)

David's Season of Waiting

Long before he sat on the throne, David found himself living as a
fugitive in the wilderness. Though anointed by the prophet Samuel
to be Israel's next king, he spent years fleeing King Saul's
relentless pursuit. By all outward appearances, David was far from
the royal seat he had been promised. Days blurred together in a
cycle of hiding in caves, strategizing escapes, and wondering why
God's timing seemed so slow. In those lonely stretches, he poured
out his heart in psalms, wrestling with despair one moment and
proclaiming trust the next. Yet, through this prolonged season,
David learned that waiting on God is never wasted time. It was

during these years that he developed the reliance, humility, and spiritual depth needed for the throne. Despite the hardship and the uncertainty, David's faith was shaped and strengthened by learning to remain steadfast, trusting that God's promises would come to fruition in the proper season.

What This Means for You

The story of David's wait offers a profound reminder that God's work often unfolds behind the scenes, beyond what we can see or understand. Waiting on the Lord does not mean idly doing nothing, nor does it imply that God has forgotten His promises. Instead, it is a call to a deeper place of trust—an invitation to remain faithful, spiritually attentive, and open to the growth that can only happen in times of stillness. Seasons of apparent inactivity can become seasons of invisible preparation, where God refines character, draws us closer to His heart, and positions us for what lies ahead. Whenever you find yourself in a waiting period—whether it's waiting on a job opportunity, healing, direction, or a relational breakthrough—remember that God's timetable is different from ours. In that space of uncertainty, learn to lean on Him and trust that He is renewing your strength for what is next.

Renewal in the Waiting

In fitness and health, we often focus on the hustle—workouts, diets, and routines designed to produce quick results. Yet physical growth and renewal also require periods of rest and recalibration, much like spiritual seasons of waiting. Muscles need time to recover after exercise, and the body benefits from planned rest days that restore energy and prevent injury. In the same way, you might enter a season when life circumstances force you to pause your usual training or modify your goals. Rather than viewing this as wasted time, see it as an essential aspect of long-term health. Use these pauses to focus on stretching, gentle movement, balanced nutrition, and mental well-being. Just as waiting on the

Lord spiritually can lead to deeper intimacy with Him, embracing restorative periods in your fitness journey can bring about renewed motivation and resilience.

Challenge

Faith Step: Consider a situation in your life where you feel in limbo—perhaps longing for a career shift, resolution in a relationship, or clarity in your calling. Instead of pressuring yourself to force a solution, dedicate this season to prayer, reflection, and the study of Scripture. Each day, meditate on a promise from God's Word that reassures you of His faithfulness. Write down moments—no matter how small—that reveal His goodness in your waiting, reminding yourself that His silence is not absence.

Physical Step: If you find yourself needing rest in your fitness journey, or if external factors have paused your usual routine, use this time to reframe how you view downtime. Incorporate gentle practices such as walks, yoga, or stretching sessions that maintain your mobility and keep you connected to your body's signals. Reflect on how both rest and waiting play key roles in renewing your physical and spiritual strength. Think of one habit—be it consistent hydration, mindful breathing, or a brief daily walk—that can help sustain and enrich your well-being until you're ready to dive back into more rigorous activity.

Waiting does not mean you are forgotten. Just as David emerged from his wilderness years prepared to lead, trust that God is using your season of stillness to shape and strengthen you in ways you may not recognize yet. Embrace the waiting, and allow your heart, mind, and body to be renewed, remembering that those who hope in the Lord will indeed find their strength restored.

13

FAITHFUL IN THE SMALL THINGS

Key Scripture: *Zechariah 4:10*

"Do not despise the day of small beginnings..." (Zechariah 4:10 paraphrased)

The Rebuilding of the Temple

After years of exile in Babylon, a remnant of God's people returned to Jerusalem to rebuild their shattered homeland. Among them was Zerubbabel, tasked with laying the foundation of a new temple—one far more modest than the glorious structure Solomon had built. Disappointment swirled around this seemingly humble start, and some who remembered the old temple mourned at how small and unimpressive the new one appeared in comparison. Yet in the midst of these doubts, God spoke through the prophet Zechariah, reminding His people not to despise the day of small beginnings. This was more than just a construction project; it

50

symbolized hope, faithfulness, and the promise that God was still with His people. Though the foundation seemed unimpressive to human eyes, the Lord took delight in every step they took to honor His name. Over time, what began as a modest foundation blossomed into a renewed place of worship, proving that God can work mightily through even the smallest starts.

What This Means for You

Zechariah's message echoes through every season of growth or change in our lives: never underestimate the power of humble beginnings. Whether you are starting a new spiritual discipline, learning a skill, or trying to rebuild a broken area of your life, the first steps might feel awkward or insignificant. However, God delights in our faithful obedience, no matter how small it may appear. The world often celebrates instant success and dramatic transformations, but lasting change usually comes in slow, steady increments. Trust that each prayer you whisper, each act of service you perform, and each new habit you cultivate is laying a foundation for deeper growth. God sees past the surface, rejoicing in your willingness to do what you can, with what you have, where you are.

Daily Small Acts

In the realm of health and fitness, it's easy to compare yourself to others or become discouraged by how far you have to go. Maybe your workout routine seems minimal, or your diet changes feel barely noticeable. Yet, just as a temple's foundation starts with one stone, building a healthier lifestyle begins with small, consistent actions. One extra glass of water, one more set of push-ups, or an extra ten minutes of walking may not look like much at first, but these humble efforts stack up over time. Rather than despising these small beginnings, celebrate them. Each small victory is a stepping stone toward larger breakthroughs, and the discipline forged in these early stages will shape your long-term success.

Challenge

Faith Step: Identify one area of your spiritual life where you need a "small beginning." Perhaps you've been meaning to pray more intentionally, read Scripture daily, or volunteer in a ministry but have felt overwhelmed by the gap between where you are and where you want to be. Commit to one small, specific action you will take each day or each week—like praying for five minutes in the morning or reading a single psalm before bed. Trust that God honors these modest starts and will grow your faith as you persist.

Physical Step: Choose one micro-change that will positively impact your health or fitness. It might be replacing one sugary beverage a day with water, doing a quick bodyweight exercise routine each morning, or adding an extra serving of vegetables to your dinner. Stick with this small habit consistently for a week or two, and track the difference you feel—both physically and mentally. Remember that over time, these seemingly insignificant changes form the bedrock of enduring transformation.

Like Zerubbabel laying that first, humble foundation stone, your small acts of faith and discipline today can become the catalysts for much bigger victories tomorrow. Embrace these beginnings, trust God's process, and allow each step to draw you closer to the vibrant, purposeful life He has in store for you.

14

PREPARE FOR MORE

Key Scripture: *2 Kings 3:16–20*

"Make this valley full of ditches… you will see neither wind nor rain, yet this valley will be filled with water." (2 Kings 3:16–17 paraphrased)

Digging Ditches in the Desert

In a desperate bid for victory, the kings of Israel, Judah, and Edom joined forces to attack Moab. But as they marched through the dry wilderness, their armies and animals ran dangerously low on water. Certain defeat loomed. In this bleak moment, the prophet Elisha delivered an unlikely command from the Lord: "Make this valley full of ditches." There was no sign of rain, no thunderclouds on the horizon, yet they were to dig ditches in the desert. Obediently, the soldiers began carving channels in the barren ground. By the next morning, water miraculously flowed through the valley, filling every trench they had prepared. What started as an inexplicable instruction became the channel of God's provision. Their readiness to dig, even without visible evidence of rain, made room for the miracle they needed.

What This Means for You

This story underscores the importance of preparing for God's blessings before they arrive. It can feel counterintuitive to set the stage for success when circumstances look unlikely or even impossible. Yet "digging ditches"—making space in faith—demonstrates trust in God's ability to provide. Perhaps there is a dream on your heart or a promise you've sensed God speaking to you, but the reality around you feels barren. Instead of waiting passively for the perfect conditions to arise, consider what actions you can take now to create room for God's future provision. Whether that means honing a skill, clearing debt, mending relationships, or dedicating more time to spiritual disciplines, your faithful preparation may be precisely what God uses to pour out His blessing.

Creating Capacity for Growth

In your fitness journey, preparing for more can be as simple as enlarging your capacity for improvement before you see immediate results. Maybe you are hoping to run faster, lift heavier, or overhaul your eating habits. You can start laying the groundwork by focusing on flexibility, perfecting your form, or learning new recipes—even if you haven't noticed a big change on the scale or in your speed yet. Like those ditches in a parched valley, these small yet concrete actions create space for future breakthroughs. Trust that the consistent groundwork you lay now—whether through mindful practice, balanced rest, or discipline in your routines—allows you to handle greater challenges and blessings down the line.

Challenge

Faith Step: Identify an area of your life where you sense God might want to do more, but you currently see no sign of progress. Ask Him how you can "dig ditches" by taking faith-filled actions in anticipation of His provision. This could include setting aside time for spiritual growth, committing to a financial plan, or serving in a new ministry where you feel called. Trust that each small act of obedience is a step toward making space for what God wants to pour into your life.

Physical Step: Think about a future fitness goal—a personal record in a race, a strength milestone, or a new level of endurance. Prepare for it by focusing on supportive habits now. If you want to run a half marathon someday, begin by steadily increasing your mileage or improving your running form. If you aim to lift heavier weights, hone your technique or add incremental, manageable increases to your routine. Picture each workout, each meal choice, and each rest day as a ditch you are digging, ready to be filled with the results you're working toward.

God invites you to prepare for more, even when your present surroundings appear barren. As you widen your capacity—in both the spiritual and physical realms—you become a ready vessel for His blessings. No matter how dry the desert may seem, trust that He can fill every channel of faith you carve out with the life-giving water of His provision.

YOU WEREN'T MADE TO STAND STILL. YOU WEREN'T CALLED JUST TO SURVIVE—YOU WERE CALLED TO STEP BOLDLY INTO THE MISSION GOD HAS SET BEFORE YOU.

YOU'VE LEARNED TO WAIT WITH FAITH. YOU'VE SEEN HOW SMALL BEGINNINGS LEAD TO GREATER THINGS. YOU'VE STOOD FIRM IN TRUST WHEN THE WAY FORWARD WASN'T CLEAR. BUT NOW—NOW IT'S TIME TO MOVE.

THE ENEMY WOULD LOVE FOR YOU TO STAY WHERE YOU ARE, TO SETTLE IN COMFORT, TO LET HESITATION ROB YOU OF YOUR CALLING. BUT GOD DIDN'T BRING YOU THIS FAR TO LEAVE YOU STANDING AT THE EDGE.

THIS IS WHERE FAITH BECOMES ACTION. THIS IS WHERE PREPARATION MEETS PURPOSE.

SO TAKE THE STEP. SPEAK THE TRUTH. FIGHT THE FIGHT. RUN THE RACE.

NOT SOMEDAY. NOT WHEN IT'S EASIER. NOW.

BECAUSE FAITH ISN'T JUST BELIEVING—IT'S MOVING. AND WHEN YOU MOVE IN FAITH, THE IMPOSSIBLE BECOMES THE INEVITABLE.

GO. STEP OUT. WALK BOLDLY INTO WHAT GOD HAS PREPARED FOR YOU. THE MISSION IS WAITING.

FROM STANDING FIRM TO STEPPING FULLY INTO THE MISSION

You've journeyed through another set of chapters—each one inviting you to dig deeper, stand stronger, wait more patiently, and prepare for greater blessings. These chapters showed you what it looks like to trust God in the stillness, to keep faith in small steps, and to make room before the miracle arrives. If you've stayed with it this far, pause and recognize that you've grown through challenges and embraced moments of quiet obedience that might not have seemed significant at first.

- You discovered the strength of standing firm, like King Jehoshaphat, trusting God to fight the battles you cannot win on your own.
- You learned how waiting on the Lord can be a season of renewal rather than stagnation, just as David's wilderness years shaped his character for kingship.
- You saw the beauty in small beginnings, realizing that even the most modest acts of faith can lay the foundation for something far greater.
- You acted in anticipation of God's future provision, digging ditches in the dry places of your life to prepare for the flow of His blessing.

Through these lessons, you've cultivated resilience, patience, and an expanded vision of what's possible when you cooperate with God's timing. But the journey isn't over.

Now, you're about to step into the final stretch, where you move from simply standing firm to walking boldly in faith. This is the moment to lean into the mission God has placed on your heart and commit to lasting transformation. Expect challenges and celebrations, breakthroughs and moments of surrender. Expect, too, a deeper resolve to keep moving forward.

Reflect & Prepare

1. **Pause and Celebrate**: Think of one insight or moment from these recent chapters that truly impacted your heart—maybe it was learning not to despise small beginnings, or realizing that your waiting season could be deeply formative. Take time to thank God for that revelation and the growth it has sparked.
2. **Name the Next Step**: Consider the place in your life where you sense God asking you to walk more boldly. Is there a dream, ministry, or relationship that needs your courage and dedication? Write it down.
3. **Commit to Ongoing Movement**: True change isn't a quick sprint; it's a faithful marathon. Ask God for the perseverance to keep going, even when your emotions dip or life gets busy. Put a practical plan in place—whether it's scheduling prayer time, setting fitness goals, or finding an accountability partner—to help you maintain forward momentum.
4.

Looking Ahead

In the final week, you'll explore what it means to step fully into your mission—to walk out the transformation you've been cultivating and stay committed for the long haul. You will be challenged to trust God on a deeper level, to move past comfort zones, and to embrace a future that reflects the growth and faith you've developed so far.

It's time to transition from standing firm to stepping out. Are you ready to put all you've learned into action and commit to an even bolder walk of faith? Let's keep going, trusting that every step you take in obedience paves the way for God's purpose in your life.

15

CALLED TO MOVE

Key scripture: *Joshua 1:1–9*

"Be strong and courageous. Do not be afraid; do not be discouraged, for the LORD your God will be with you wherever you go." (Joshua 1:9 paraphrased)

God's Charge to Joshua

Moses, the great leader of Israel, had died, and the mantle of leadership passed to Joshua. Standing at the threshold of the Promised Land, the people of Israel felt both anticipation and uncertainty. They had witnessed God's miraculous provision in the wilderness, but now a new challenge loomed: occupying a land filled with formidable obstacles and enemies. In this moment of transition, God delivered a resounding charge to Joshua: "Be strong and courageous." He promised His abiding presence and reminded Joshua of the covenant made with Moses—that every place they set foot would belong to them, so long as they walked in obedience. These words were more than just a pep talk; they were a divine commissioning, a statement that Joshua's next steps would have a profound impact not only on himself but on the entire nation he was called to lead. Bolstered by God's assurance, Joshua moved forward, guiding Israel across the Jordan River and into an uncharted future that required faith, bravery, and steadfast commitment to God's Word.

What This Means for You

Like Joshua standing on the edge of the Promised Land, you are called to move forward in faith, carrying a mission that extends beyond your personal benefit. It can be intimidating to leave familiar ground, whether that's a comfortable routine, a particular career path, or a mindset of self-doubt. Yet God often invites His people to go where they haven't gone before, promising His presence and urging them to be strong and courageous. Embracing this call means recognizing that your steps of obedience can have a ripple effect on the people around you—family, friends, your community, or even those you have yet to meet. God equips you not just for self-improvement, but for a larger kingdom purpose. Whenever you find yourself hesitating, remember that God's assurances to Joshua apply to you as well: "I will never leave you nor forsake you."

Moving for a Bigger Purpose

In the same way that Joshua's call was bigger than his personal journey, your health and wellness pursuits can influence more than just your own life. When you prioritize regular exercise, balanced nutrition, and rest, you model a lifestyle of stewardship for those around you—children, friends, or coworkers who may be encouraged by your example. This doesn't mean your journey will be without obstacles; you might face temptations, plateaus, or discouragement. But just like Joshua had to trust God's direction in uncharted territory, you can trust that each new step you take—

whether it's trying a new workout, learning healthier habits, or seeking accountability—serves a greater purpose than merely looking or feeling better. It becomes a testimony of what God can do when you surrender every aspect of your life, including your physical well-being, to His guidance.

Challenge

Faith Step: Identify one area in which you sense God urging you to move forward for the sake of something larger than yourself—perhaps serving in a new ministry, reaching out to someone in need, or sharing your faith story more boldly. Ask God for the same courage He gave Joshua, and take a practical step toward that calling this week. Write it down, pray over it, and trust God to go with you.

Physical Step: Reflect on how your health journey might bless others. Could you invite a friend or family member to join you for a walk, share healthy recipes with someone trying to improve their diet, or start a small exercise group at church or work? Think about a meaningful way to extend your wellness habits to benefit others, and commit to putting that idea into action.

Like Joshua, stand on the brink of new territory with confidence. Every move you make in faith, every act of courage, and every moment of obedience positions you to carry out the mission God has set before you. Like Joshua, stand on the brink of new territory with confidence. He has called you not just for your own growth, but so that His presence and purpose might radiate through your life into the world around you.

16

DO NOT FEAR

Key Scripture: *Isaiah 43:1–2*

"Do not fear, for I have redeemed you; I have summoned you by name; you are mine. When you pass through the waters, I will be with you..." (Isaiah 43:1–2 paraphrased)

Israel's Assurance of God's Presence

During a time of uncertainty and exile, the people of Israel clung to the promise that they were still God's chosen ones. Though they had lost their homeland and found themselves in unfamiliar territory, God spoke through the prophet Isaiah to deliver a resounding message: "Do not fear, for I have redeemed you." These were not merely comforting words; they were a divine declaration that the Creator had not abandoned His people. Israel had endured harsh bondage and disheartening setbacks, yet the

Lord reminded them of His unfailing presence and unwavering claim on their lives. He promised to walk with them through the torrent of challenges and the fires of adversity, ensuring that they would not be consumed. In these few verses, God boldly reaffirmed His covenant, declaring that no matter how threatening their circumstances appeared, He would remain their steadfast protector and guide.

What This Means for You

Fear has a way of shrinking our world. It can keep us from stepping out in faith or fully embracing a calling that God has placed on our hearts. Yet the same message God gave to Israel holds true for anyone who struggles with doubts and anxieties: "Do not fear… you are mine." When you belong to the Lord, no trial or unknown future can separate you from His care. This assurance empowers you to move forward in boldness, knowing that you are never alone. Each time you confront fear—whether it's the fear of rejection, failure, or the unknown—you affirm the reality that you have been redeemed by One who calls you by name. Your identity in Christ transcends any obstacle you face. Embracing this truth frees you to take risks in obedience, to trust beyond what you can see, and to refuse a life defined by worry.

Overcoming Fear in Your Journey

In your physical health and fitness journey, fear often masks itself in excuses or self-doubt—"I'm too old," "I'll never stick to it," "What if I fail again?" Yet God's words in Isaiah 43 remind you that your worth and potential lie not in your perceived limitations, but in His redeeming power. When you choose to challenge yourself— maybe by starting a new workout plan, running a mile further, or cutting back on unhealthy habits—you acknowledge that fear does not have the final say. Each small victory, every new record or healthier meal, testifies that God's strength is at work in your body as well as your spirit. Rather than letting fear paralyze you, let it serve as a reminder to lean deeper into the One who equips you for every good work, including caring for the body He has entrusted to you.

Challenge

Faith Step: Identify a specific fear that has been holding you back from saying "yes" to God's call—whether it's serving in a certain area, pursuing a dream, or reconciling a broken relationship. Write that fear down. Then, pray through Isaiah 43:1–2, inviting the Lord to meet you in that anxiety with His reassurance and strength. Take at least one tangible step to move beyond your fear—such as reaching out for guidance, making a phone call you've been avoiding, or signing up for that ministry you've been considering.

Physical Step: Consider an area in your fitness or wellness routine where fear keeps you stuck—maybe it's attending a group class, trying a challenging exercise, or altering a long-held eating habit. Make a commitment to step outside your comfort zone. Sign up for that class, experiment with a new workout, or talk to a nutritionist. Let each action be a declaration that fear does not control you, and trust that God is with you, step by step.

From Isaiah's words to the exiles in Babylon to your own challenges today, God's invitation remains the same: do not fear. He has called you by name, and you belong to Him. Let this assurance push you past the boundaries that once confined you, so you can walk boldly into the life and mission for which you were redeemed.

17

EMPOWERED TO ACT

Key Scripture: *Joel 2:28–29*

"I will pour out my Spirit on all people... Even on my servants, both men and women, I will pour out my Spirit in those days." (Joel 2:28–29 paraphrased)

The Promise of God's Spirit

Through the prophet Joel, God spoke to a nation that had endured a devastating locust plague and profound spiritual decline. In the midst of warning and lament, however, there was a spark of hope: a promise that one day, God would pour out His Spirit in a way never seen before. This wasn't reserved for kings or prophets alone—everyone, from the youngest child to the oldest servant, would experience the power and presence of God firsthand. The Spirit would stir dreams and visions, igniting hearts with divine purpose and empowering ordinary men and women to do extraordinary things. Centuries later, on the Day of Pentecost, this promise was fulfilled in a dramatic display of tongues of fire and transformed lives, confirming that Joel's words were not confined to an ancient era but continue to echo into every generation of believers.

What This Means for You

The good news is that you don't have to muster the strength for spiritual growth, bold faith, or consistent obedience on your own. God is not an aloof bystander, watching from afar as you struggle. Instead, the same Spirit who revived a devastated nation and empowered the early church is available to empower you today. Whether you feel weak, overwhelmed, or underqualified, God offers His Spirit to supply the courage, wisdom, and perseverance you lack. This is not a temporary motivational boost; it's a life-giving relationship with the divine presence that renews you from the inside out. If there's a specific mission, ministry, or challenge in your life that seems daunting, remember that God never intended for you to tackle it in your own strength. His Spirit within you can transform fear into action and uncertainty into unwavering faith.

Partnering with God's Power

Your physical well-being can also be a place where you witness the Spirit's empowering presence. While discipline and hard work are vital, there's a deeper dimension available when you invite God into your health journey. Think of the Spirit as the "wind in your sails," energizing your efforts and correcting your course when you lose motivation or direction. Have you ever felt a nudge to keep going when everything in you wants to quit, or found clarity amidst confusion about your next step? Such moments can be hints that God's Spirit is actively guiding you. Whether you're striving to break old habits, recover from an injury, or simply maintain a routine, asking the Holy Spirit for help can bridge the gap between your best efforts and God's transforming power.

Challenge

Faith Step: Reflect on a task or calling in your life that seems beyond your capabilities—something you're hesitant to tackle because you feel inadequate. Commit this to prayer, asking the Holy Spirit to fill you afresh with strength, courage, and wisdom. Take one action step this week that demonstrates your willingness to depend on His power, whether it's volunteering for a ministry, having a spiritual conversation with a friend, or stepping into a leadership role you've been avoiding.

Physical Step: Look for opportunities to practice inviting the Spirit's help in your health or fitness goals. Before a workout or any physical challenge, pause for a moment and ask God to guide your efforts. If you hit a hurdle—whether it's a gym plateau or a dietary struggle—pray for fresh motivation and resilience. Notice how your mindset and perseverance shift when you intentionally remember you're not alone in these goals.

However overwhelming life's demands may appear, remember that God has poured out His Spirit to empower you. As you learn to rely on His presence in both spiritual endeavors and practical challenges, you'll find that you can move forward with a new courage and effectiveness that surpass your own natural abilities. You have a divine helper who stands ready to guide your steps, strengthen your resolve, and help you become all that He's called you to be.

18

PRESS THROUGH THE OBSTACLES

Key Scripture: *Daniel 6*

"When Daniel learned that the decree had been published, he went home... three times a day he got down on his knees and prayed, giving thanks to his God..." (Daniel 6:10 paraphrased)

Daniel in the Lion's Den

Daniel was a man of steadfast integrity, promoted to a high position in the kingdom of Darius. His excellence and devotion to God sparked jealousy among other officials, who devised a law forbidding prayer to anyone but the king. Despite the threat of death, Daniel continued his daily practice of prayer, refusing to break faith with the Lord he served. His enemies seized the opportunity, reporting Daniel's actions and insisting he be thrown into a den of ravenous lions. Overnight, Daniel remained in that perilous place, surrounded by real danger, yet he emerged unharmed the next morning, safeguarded by an angel who silenced the lions' jaws. This miraculous deliverance not only saved Daniel's life but also led King Darius to acknowledge the power of Daniel's God. In the face of a formidable obstacle—one that could have cost him everything—Daniel's unwavering faith stood as a testimony to God's sustaining power.

What This Means for You

Daniel's story challenges us to maintain our commitment to God even when the stakes are high. Obstacles in life may not always look like literal lions, but they can feel just as insurmountable. Fear, opposition, or disappointment can roar loudly, tempting us to compromise or step away from what we know is right. Yet Daniel's example demonstrates that faithful perseverance often paves the way for divine intervention. Whether you're facing a financial crisis, dealing with relationship conflict, or wrestling with spiritual doubt, God remains present in the midst of the turmoil. He can shut the mouths of your "lions," turning potential defeat into a powerful display of His protection and grace. What matters is your willingness to hold onto faith, praying consistently, and trusting that God is able to deliver you—even if the outcome isn't what you first expect.

Overcoming Setbacks and Discouragement

Physical health and fitness goals are rarely a straight line. Injuries, plateaus, busy schedules, and self-doubt can all feel like lions blocking your path. You might find yourself discouraged when progress stalls or frustration mounts. In these moments, remember Daniel's persistence in prayer and devotion. Allow that same steadfast mindset to shape how you approach obstacles. Rather than giving up or compromising, adjust your plan, seek wise counsel, or incorporate rest and recovery as part of your regimen. Pressing through physical challenges might involve patience and creativity, but it also requires the same ingredient that carried Daniel through his trial: unwavering commitment. Ultimately, it's not just about reaching a fitness milestone—it's about building the habit of perseverance that honors both your body and the God who gave it to you.

Challenge

Faith Step: Identify a "lion's den" in your life—a situation where fear or opposition threatens your peace or convictions. Like Daniel, commit to consistent prayer in that area. If you've been tempted to compromise, ask God for renewed faith and the courage to hold firm. Jot down a plan for how you'll pray and lean on Scripture daily, inviting God to intervene in ways that strengthen your trust in Him.

Physical Step: Think about a fitness obstacle you've been avoiding or an ongoing issue that's preventing you from hitting your goals. Pinpoint one practical strategy to address it—a new workout approach, a consult with a professional (such as a trainer or physical therapist), or a schedule adjustment to ensure consistency. Share this plan with someone who can support you, and make a concrete commitment to persevere through the challenge.

Daniel's victory in the lions' den reminds us that *faith is not just an internal feeling; it's an active choice* to keep trusting and obeying God, regardless of the cost. As you face your own obstacles— whether spiritual, relational, or physical—stand firm in faith and let God show His strength on your behalf. When you remain steadfast, He is more than capable of carrying you through any challenge that stands in your way.

19

THE REWARD FOR PERSEVERANCE

Key Scripture: *Deuteronomy 28*

"If you fully obey the LORD your God and carefully follow all His commands… all these blessings will come on you and accompany you…" (Deuteronomy 28:1–2 paraphrased)

Blessings for Obedience

As Moses prepared the Israelites to enter the Promised Land, he laid out a clear choice in Deuteronomy 28: obey God's commands and receive His abundant blessings, or disregard His ways and invite consequences. This was not a transactional deal but rather a covenantal promise rooted in God's deep desire to see His people flourish in the land He had promised them. Obedience would bring favor in their cities and fields, in their families and livestock, in their coming and going. The Israelites, who had wandered in the desert for decades, now stood at the brink of a new chapter, reminded that their faithfulness would shape their future. Even

72

though challenges lay ahead, their determination to persevere in obedience would usher them into a life of tangible provision and spiritual wholeness.

What This Means for You

The rewards promised to Israel reflect God's heart toward anyone who commits to faithful living. While the specific agricultural blessings of ancient times may look different today, the principle remains: God honors perseverance and obedience. This doesn't mean you'll never face hardship; rather, it means that your steadfast pursuit of God's ways positions you to receive His favor—spiritually, relationally, and sometimes even materially. The journey of obedience can be long and demanding, but Scripture consistently reveals that God sees and rewards those who hold fast to Him. When you serve faithfully, pray diligently, or persevere in moral integrity, you are participating in a covenant relationship with the Lord. You can trust that He will meet you there with goodness, provision, and purpose, even if His timing or methods aren't exactly what you expect.

Reaping the Benefits of Consistency

In health and fitness, consistent perseverance pays off as well. It's easy to start a new exercise routine or diet with enthusiasm, only to let discouragement derail you at the first sign of a plateau. However, just like Israel on the verge of the Promised Land, you stand to gain significant "blessings" by sticking to the course—improved stamina, better mental health, and a sense of accomplishment that spills over into other areas of life. These physical rewards mirror the spiritual reality that faithfulness leads to fruitfulness. Every mile run, every workout completed, every healthy meal prepared becomes a seed planted in good soil, eventually yielding the harvest of a stronger body and increased well-being.

Challenge

Faith Step: Consider one area of obedience in your spiritual life that could use a renewed commitment—maybe it's praying regularly for someone who's wronged you, serving in a ministry you've been hesitant to join, or obeying God in a specific personal conviction. Reflect on Deuteronomy 28, and ask God to help you persevere, trusting that He sees and rewards even the smallest steps of obedience.

Physical Step: Identify a point in your fitness routine or health journey where you often give up or lose focus. Perhaps you struggle to exercise consistently, skip meals, or let stress sabotage your diet. This week, pledge to push through that critical moment of weakness or discouragement. Write down what action you'll take—whether it's committing to a set time for workouts or prepping meals in advance—and ask at least one person to hold you accountable.

Faithful movement—both in spirit and body—positions you for blessings that exceed what you might initially imagine. The history of God's covenant with Israel stands as a reminder that obedience is neither futile nor empty; it's an invitation to experience the fullness of God's favor. As you persevere, keep your eyes on the One who rewards those who earnestly seek Him, confident that your diligence will not be in vain.

20

FINISHING STRONG

Key Scripture: *2 Chronicles 31:20–21*

"Hezekiah did what was good and right and faithful before the LORD his God. In everything that he undertook… he sought his God and worked wholeheartedly. And so he prospered." (2 Chronicles 31:20–21 paraphrased)

Hezekiah's Commitment

Hezekiah became king during a turbulent period in Judah's history. The people had grown lax in their worship, neglecting the temple and sliding into idolatry. Rather than caving to apathy or following the example of his compromised predecessors, Hezekiah chose to restore true worship. He reopened the temple doors, cleansed and consecrated the priests, and called the people back to God. It wasn't just a one-time push—Hezekiah consistently pursued reforms that honored the Lord, reorganizing the priesthood and reinstituting faithful practices throughout the land. Under his leadership, Judah experienced a season of revival and blessing. When crises arose—such as the threat from the Assyrian army—Hezekiah faced them with unwavering faith, praying wholeheartedly for deliverance. Although his reign wasn't free from trials, he finished strong by maintaining the same devotion to God from his early reforms until his final days, demonstrating that true faithfulness involves carrying through, even as challenges accumulate over time.

What This Means for You

Hezekiah's story illustrates that finishing strong requires more than a strong start or an isolated moment of commitment. It's about perseverance—a day-in, day-out dedication that endures until the end. Maybe you've experienced seasons in which you began with enthusiasm but grew weary halfway through—whether in spiritual disciplines, personal goals, or service to others. Hezekiah's example reminds you that faithfulness is sustained by continually seeking God, allowing Him to renew your resolve. It's less about perfection and more about wholehearted devotion, even when faced with pressures and setbacks. Wherever you are in your journey—whether just beginning a new habit of prayer, nearing a milestone in your career, or leading others in a ministry—God honors the individual who stays the course. The real victory is not in merely starting well, but in maintaining that spirit of obedience and trust to the very end.

Seeing It Through

Your health journey, like Hezekiah's reforms, requires consistent dedication rather than periodic bursts of energy. Perhaps you began exercising with gusto or switched to healthier eating habits, only to find your motivation waning as the novelty wore off. This final chapter challenges you to keep going, to finish what you started. Even if progress seems slow, remember that lasting change isn't a sprint; it's a marathon. Whether you're recovering from an injury, juggling a hectic schedule, or simply battling the inertia that comes with routine, a "finish strong" mindset pushes you to stay faithful to the process. You may need to adjust strategies, seek accountability, or learn new approaches—but the key is not giving up halfway. Each healthy choice, every workout session, and each moment of discipline is a step toward completing what you set out to do.

Challenge

Faith Step: Look back on a spiritual commitment you made—maybe at the start of these chapters or at some other point in your life—and evaluate how it's going. Ask yourself: Have I grown tired or allowed distractions to derail me? Pray for renewed zeal and ask God to help you finish strong. If needed, set a fresh goal or recommit to a spiritual discipline, such as regular time in Scripture or consistent church involvement.

Physical Step: Identify a health or fitness plan you began but struggled to maintain. Reassess it honestly, adjusting if necessary to fit your current season of life. Then, create a clear, short-term goal (for the next week or month) and a longer-term vision (for the next few months). Share these with someone you trust, asking them to encourage you and hold you to your commitments. Let this be your declaration that you will see it through, not out of mere willpower, but by depending on God's strength and honoring the body He's given you.

Scripture affirms that God "strengthens the weary and increases the power of the weak." He longs to see you finish the races you start—both spiritually and physically. Like Hezekiah, work wholeheartedly at whatever the Lord entrusts to you, and trust that He will bring you to a strong and faithful finish.

21

KEEP MOVING FORWARD

Key Scripture: *Habakkuk 3:17–19*

"Though the fig tree does not bud and there are no grapes on the vines… yet I will rejoice in the LORD, I will be joyful in God my Savior." (Habakkuk 3:17–18 paraphrased)

Habakkuk's Unshakable Trust

In a time of national crisis and impending judgment, the prophet Habakkuk wrestled with tough questions about God's justice and timing. He saw corruption within his own people and imminent threats from foreign powers. Initially perplexed by God's plan, Habakkuk engaged in earnest dialogue with the Lord, seeking answers and expressing his frustrations. Yet by the final chapter, his lament transformed into a profound declaration of trust. Even if circumstances remained dire—if harvests failed, livestock disappeared, and hope seemed thin—Habakkuk resolved to rejoice in the Lord. It was not a shallow optimism but a determined faith that God would sustain him, come what may. This final posture of the prophet underscores that sometimes the greatest victory is to stand firm in hope, continuing forward even when visible results are scarce.

What This Means for You

Habakkuk's resolution points to a reality that echoes throughout Scripture: walking with God isn't a short-term sprint but a lifelong journey of trust. You may have reached the end of these 21 days of spiritual and physical focus, but that doesn't mean your quest for transformation should end. True growth and endurance come when you continue seeking, praying, and obeying—even when immediate results aren't evident. Like Habakkuk, you may not always see the fruit you anticipate. Circumstances might even worsen before they improve. But choosing to rejoice in God, no matter what, sets you on a path of steadfast faith that transcends fleeting changes or short-lived accomplishments. When your energy wanes or obstacles loom large, remember that your ultimate strength and security come from the Lord, not from momentary victories.

Building a Lifestyle, Not a 21-Day Sprint

Just as spiritual growth is a lifelong pursuit, your health journey is also meant to continue beyond any single plan or challenge. Perhaps you began these chapters hoping to reset your routine or overcome a lingering hurdle in your fitness. Think of this final day as a launching pad for a longer, more sustainable commitment. Habakkuk's unyielding trust in God, even when the fields were barren, reminds you that transformation is about faithfulness rather than quick fixes. When results don't come as fast as you'd like—if the scale doesn't budge right away, or your endurance doesn't skyrocket overnight—staying the course is what truly matters. Each day is another opportunity to refine habits, train your body, and honor God by caring for the life He's given you.

Challenge

Faith Step: Reflect on these 21 chapters and identify a key lesson or theme that resonated with you. Maybe it was learning to step out in faith despite fear, or discovering the power of standing firm in a waiting season. Write a brief commitment statement about how you plan to continue integrating that truth into your everyday life. Consider sharing this commitment with a mentor or close friend who can keep you accountable as you move forward.

Physical Step: Instead of ending your health and fitness goals now, craft a simple roadmap for the next few weeks or months. This might include incremental goals—like increasing your running mileage, trying a new workout routine, or consistently preparing nutritious meals. Schedule a check-in with yourself or a friend 30 days from now to evaluate your progress. Let this new timeline serve as a reminder that your health journey is ongoing, not confined to a short challenge.

Whether in your spiritual walk or your physical endeavors, "finishing" these pages should mark the beginning of a deeper, more sustained pursuit of growth. Like Habakkuk, choose to trust God's goodness in every circumstance, confident that He sustains you beyond any 21-day window. As you keep moving forward— step by step, day by day—know that God's grace empowers you to persevere, and His presence accompanies you every mile of the journey ahead.

CONCLUSION

A LIFELONG JOURNEY OF FAITH AND ACTION

You've just completed a 21-chapter journey—one that invited you to move forward in faith, care for your physical well-being, and trust God in every season. Throughout these pages, you've explored stories of ordinary people who took extraordinary steps, endured wilderness seasons, stood firm in the face of opposition, and witnessed miracles that only God could perform. You've seen how small beginnings matter, how waiting can refine rather than stall you, and how each move of obedience is a ditch dug in anticipation of God's blessing.

But more important than any single concept or strategy is the overarching reminder that this journey doesn't end with the final page. True transformation—spiritual, physical, and otherwise—is a process, not a quick milestone to check off. In the same way that the Israelites had to keep moving, keep worshiping, and keep growing even after crossing the Red Sea, you, too, are called to continue walking forward in faith.

Keep returning to the truths you've uncovered here:

- God's promises still stand, even when life's circumstances feel uncertain.

- Consistency and small acts of faith forge lasting change, long after an initial burst of motivation.
- Perseverance matters: whether you're overcoming a spiritual hurdle or pushing through a health plateau, your steadfast effort honors God and shapes your character.
- You don't walk alone. The Holy Spirit is an ever-present helper, and a community of fellow believers can encourage you when your own strength feels lacking.

Consider reviewing these chapters again when you face a new challenge or find your motivation waning. Let the stories of Scripture, the reflection questions, and the action steps serve as both a compass and a lifeline. And remember: the same God who guided Abraham, parted the Red Sea for Moses, empowered Joshua to be strong and courageous, and strengthened Daniel in the lions' den is at work in your life today.

The path ahead is still unfolding, but take heart—each day is another opportunity to grow, to trust, to love, and to serve. Press on with hope, knowing that as you keep moving, both in body and spirit, you'll continue discovering more of God's presence, purpose, and power. May this be only the beginning of a deeper, richer experience of life lived hand-in-hand with the One who calls you forward.

ABOUT THE AUTHOR

Michelle Frase is a passionate follower of Christ whose heart for spiritual growth and holistic wellness inspired her to create this 21-day journey. Drawing on her love for Scripture and her commitment to living an active, balanced life, Michelle weaves biblical truths together with practical health insights to encourage others on their own paths of transformation. Through her writing and speaking, she aims to help believers discover that caring for the body and nurturing the spirit are deeply interwoven parts of a thriving faith.

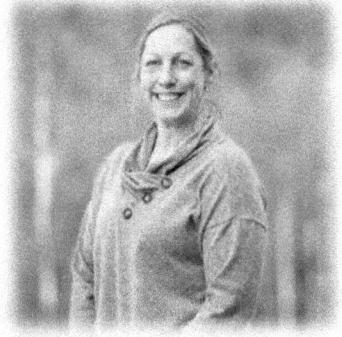

Michelle's enthusiasm for the Old Testament shines throughout her work. She believes these ancient stories offer timeless wisdom, serving as a tangible testimony from the heroes of faith who have gone before us—"the great cloud of witnesses," as Hebrews 12:1 describes—cheering us on to run our race with perseverance. From the parting of the Red Sea to Nehemiah's rebuilding efforts, she demonstrates a gift for connecting the grit and grace of biblical narratives with the real-life challenges faced by readers today.

In addition to her passion for writing and teaching, Michelle directs a faith-based gym and fitness center organized by her church, a place she affectionately calls "the church the other six days of the week." There, she helps people integrate physical exercise with spiritual growth, creating a community where members can pursue holistic health grounded in biblical principles.

Whether she's leading small-group discussions, hosting fitness challenges, or writing, Michelle's deepest desire is to see people embrace the abundant life God has promised—one in which movement, discipline, and faith work hand-in-hand. Her approachable style and genuine compassion stem from her own journey of relying on God's strength through both trials and triumphs. She prays that this book will serve as a spark that propels you closer to Jesus, inviting you to keep moving forward in faith—long after Day 21.

A Personal Invitation to Salvation

Hey friend,

I don't know where you are in life right now—what struggles you're facing, what questions you're wrestling with—but I do know this: **God sees you. He loves you. And He wants a real relationship with you.**

This isn't about religion or trying to be "good enough." It's about receiving a gift—one that Jesus already paid for because He loves you that much. If you've ever wondered how to truly know God and have eternal life, here's the simple truth:

1. You Need a Savior

Let's be real—we've all messed up. We've all sinned, fallen short, and tried to do life our own way. That sin separates us from God, and no amount of good deeds can fix it.

Romans 3:23 – "For all have sinned and fall short of the glory of God."
Romans 6:23 – "For the wages of sin is death, but the gift of God is eternal life in Christ Jesus our Lord."

Without Jesus, we're stuck in our sin. But the good news? **God didn't leave us there.**

2. Jesus Came for You

God loves you so much that He made a way for you to be saved. He sent Jesus—His own Son—to take your place. Jesus willingly died for your sins, was buried, and three days later, He rose again. He defeated death so you could have life.

John 3:16 – "For God so loved the world that He gave His one and only Son, that whoever believes in Him shall not perish but have eternal life."
☒ *Romans 5:8* – "But God demonstrates His own love for us in this: While we were still sinners, Christ died for us."

This is how much **you** matter to Him.

3. Say Yes to Jesus

This isn't about just believing in your head—it's about trusting Jesus with your whole heart. Salvation is a choice. It's a decision to stop running, stop trying to do life alone, and surrender everything to the One who created you.

Romans 10:9 – "If you declare with your mouth, 'Jesus is Lord,' and believe in your heart that God raised Him from the dead, you will be saved."

That's it. It's not about earning anything—it's about receiving what Jesus has already done for you.

4. Receive His Gift

Salvation is a **gift**—you can't work for it, you can't buy it, and you definitely can't earn it. All you can do is say **yes**.

Ephesians 2:8-9 – "For it is by grace you have been saved, through faith—and this is not from yourselves, it is the gift of God—not by works, so that no one can boast."

Jesus is offering you new life—right now. Will you take it?

5. Pray & Surrender Your Life to Jesus

If you're ready to follow Jesus, you don't need fancy words or a perfect prayer—just an honest heart. If you're not sure what to say, you can pray something like this:

"Jesus, I know that I am a sinner and I need Your forgiveness. I believe You died on the cross for me and rose again. I turn from my old life and ask You to come into my heart. Be my Lord and Savior. I surrender my life to You. Help me follow You from this day forward. Thank You for saving me. In Jesus' name, Amen."

If you just prayed that prayer and meant it, **you are saved.** Not because of anything you did, but because Jesus made the way. Welcome to the family of God!

6. Keep Walking with God

Salvation isn't the finish line—it's the beginning of an incredible journey. Find a Bible-believing church, start reading the Bible (I recommend starting with the book of John), and surround yourself with people who will encourage you in your faith.

2 Corinthians 5:17 – "Therefore, if anyone is in Christ, the new creation has come: The old has gone, the new is here!"

You don't have to figure this out alone. **God is with you, and I'm cheering you on.** Keep moving forward—one step at a time. You were made for this.

www.ingramcontent.com/pod-product-compliance
Lightning Source LLC
Chambersburg PA
CBHW052101270326
41931CB00012B/2847